Aids to the Examination of the Peripheral Nervous System

Baillière Tindall

LONDON PHILADELPHIA TORONTO
SYDNEY TOKYO

Baillière Tindall   24–28 Oval Road,
W. B. Saunders   London NW1 7DX.

West Washington Square
Philadelphia, PA 19105, USA

1 Goldthorne Avenue
Toronto, Ontario M8Z 5T9, Canada

ABP Australia Ltd, 44–50 Waterloo Road
North Ryde, NSW 2113, Australia

Harcourt Brace Jovanovich Japan Inc.,
Ichibancho Central Building, 22–1 Ichibancho
Chiyoda-ku, Tokyo 102, Japan

This edition first published 1986
Reprinted 1988

Printed and bound in Great Britain at
The Alden Press, Oxford

British Library Cataloguing in Publication Data

Aids to the examination of the peripheral nervous system.
   —[New ed.]
   1. Nerves, Peripheral—Diseases—Diagnosis
   616.8'70754   RC409

ISBN 0–7020–1165–7

Preface

In 1940 Dr. George Riddoch was Consultant Neurologist to the Army. He realised the necessity of providing centres to deal with peripheral nerve injuries during the war. In collaboration with Professor Learmonth, Professor of Surgery at the University of Edinburgh, peripheral nerve injury centres were established at Gogarburn near Edinburgh and at Killearn near Glasgow. Professor Learmonth wished to have an illustrated guide on peripheral nerve injuries for the use of surgeons working in general hospitals. In collaboration with Dr. Ritchie Russell, a few photographs demonstrating the testing of individual muscles were taken in 1941, but Dr. Ritchie Russell returned to Oxford in 1942 and was replaced by Dr. McArdle as Neurologist to Scottish Command. The photographs were completed by Dr. McArdle at Gogarburn with the help of the Department of Medical Illustration at the University of Edinburgh. About twenty copies in loose-leaf form were circulated to surgeons in Scotland.

In 1943 Professor Learmonth and Dr. Riddoch added the diagrams illustrating the innervation of muscles by various peripheral nerves modified from Pitres and Testut, and also the diagrams of cutaneous sensory distributions and dermatomes. This work was published by the Medical Research Council in 1943 as *Aids to the Investigation of Peripheral Nerve Injuries* (War Memorandum No. 7). It became a standard work and over the next thirty years many thousands of copies were printed.

It was thoroughly revised between 1972 and 1975 with new photographs and many new diagrams and was republished under the title *Aids to the Examination of the Peripheral Nervous System* (Memorandum No. 45), reflecting the wide use made of this booklet by students and practitioners and its more extensive use in clinical neurology, which was rather different from the war time emphasis on nerve injuries.

In 1984 the Medical Research Council transferred responsibility for this publication to the Guarantors of *Brain* for whom this new edition has been prepared. Modifications have been made to some of the diagrams and a new diagram of the lumbosacral plexus has been included.

The Editorial Committee for the
Guarantors of *Brain* 1985

Acknowledgements

Figs. 1, 2, 6, 7, 10, 11, 21, 23, 29, 30, 31, 32, 34, 35, 37 and 40 have been reproduced with permission from the Institute of Neurology, The National Hospital for Nervous Diseases

Figs. 3, 4, 5, 8, 9, 12, 13, 14, 15, 16, 17, 18, 19, 20, 22, 24, 25, 26, 27, 28, 33, 36, 38, 39, 41, 42, 43, 44, 46, 47, 48, 49, 50, 51, 52, 53, 54, 55, 56, 57, 58, 59, 60, 61, 62, 63, 64, 65, 66, 67, 87, 88, 89 and 90 have been reproduced with permission from Guy's Hospital Medical School.

We are grateful to Patricia Archer for the drawings of the brachial and lumbosacral plexuses and for redrawing some of the other figures.

Contents

Introduction

This atlas is intended as a guide to the examination of patients with lesions of peripheral nerves and nerve roots.

These examinations should, if possible, be conducted in a quiet room where patient and examiner will be free from distraction. For both motor and sensory testing it is important that the patient should first be warm. The nature and object of the tests should be explained to the patient so that his interest and co-operation are secured. If either shows signs of fatigue the session should be discontinued and resumed later.

Motor testing

A muscle may act as a *prime mover*, as a *fixator*, as an *antagonist*, or as a *synergist*. Thus, flexor carpi ulnaris acts as a *prime mover* when it flexes and adducts the wrist; as a *fixator* when it immobilises the pisiform bone during contraction of the abductor digiti minimi; as an *antagonist* when it resists extension of the wrist; and as a *synergist* when the digits, but not the wrists, are extended.

As far as possible the action of each muscle should be observed separately and a note made of those in which power has been retained as well as of those that are weak or paralysed. It is usual to examine the power of a muscle in relation to the movement of a single joint. It has long been customary to use a 0 to 5 scale for recording muscle power, but it is now generally recognised that subdivision of grade 4 may be helpful.

0   No contraction
1   Flicker or trace of contraction
2   Active movement, with gravity eliminated
3   Active movement against gravity
4   Active movement against gravity and resistance
5   Normal power

Grades 4−, 4 and 4+, may be used to indicate movement against slight, moderate and strong resistance respectively.

The models employed in this work were not chosen because they showed unusual muscular development; but the ease with which the contraction of muscles is identified varies with the build of the patient, and it is essential that the examiner should both look for and endeavour to feel the contraction of an accessible muscle and/or the movement of its tendon. In most of the illustrations the optimum point for palpation has been marked.

Muscles have been arranged in the order of the origin of their motor supply from nerve trunks, which is convenient in many examinations. Usually only

1

one method of testing each muscle is shown but, where necessary, multiple illustrations have been included if a muscle has more than one important action. The examiner should apply the tests as they are illustrated, because the techniques shown will eliminate many of the traps for the inexperienced provided by 'trick' movements. It should be noted that each of the methods used tests, as a rule, the action of muscles at a single joint.

The usual nerve supply to each muscle is stated in the captions, and the spinal segments from which it is derived, the more important of the latter being printed in heavy type. Tables showing limb muscles arranged according to their supply by individual nerve roots and peripheral nerves are to be found on pages 60–61.

Sensory testing

The patient is first asked to outline the area of sensory abnormality; this can be a useful guide to the detailed examination. Light touch should be tested by touches with something soft such as cotton wool, working from the insensitive towards the sensitive area. If the area of sensory abnormality is hypersensitive the direction is reversed. The area delineated is marked by a continuous line. For testing superficial pain a sharp pin is best and again — unless there is apparent hypersensitivity (hyperpathia) — the stimuli are applied first to the analgesic area, working outwards. The area is outlined by a series of dots. The timing of the stimuli should be irregular so that the patient does not know when to expect the next touch or pinprick.

It may also be important to test two-point discrimination on the fingers, joint position sense and, on occasion, deep pressure sense.

The area of skin supplied by any one nerve or nerve root varies from patient to patient, as exemplified by the median (Fig. 75) and ulnar (Fig. 76) nerves. The areas shown in the diagrams are the usual ones.

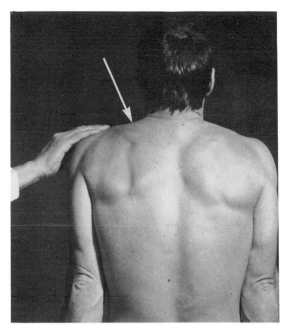

Fig. 1 Trapezius (Spinal accessory nerve and C3, C4)
The patient is elevating the shoulder against resistance. *Arrow:* the thick upper part of the muscle can be seen and felt.

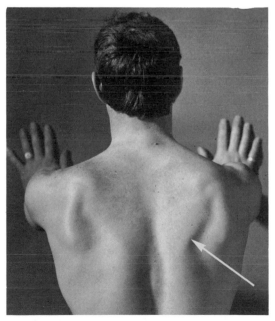

Fig. 2 Trapezius (Spinal accessory nerve and C3, C4)
The patient is pushing the palms of the hands hard against a wall with the elbows fully extended. *Arrow:* the lower fibres of trapezius can be seen and felt.

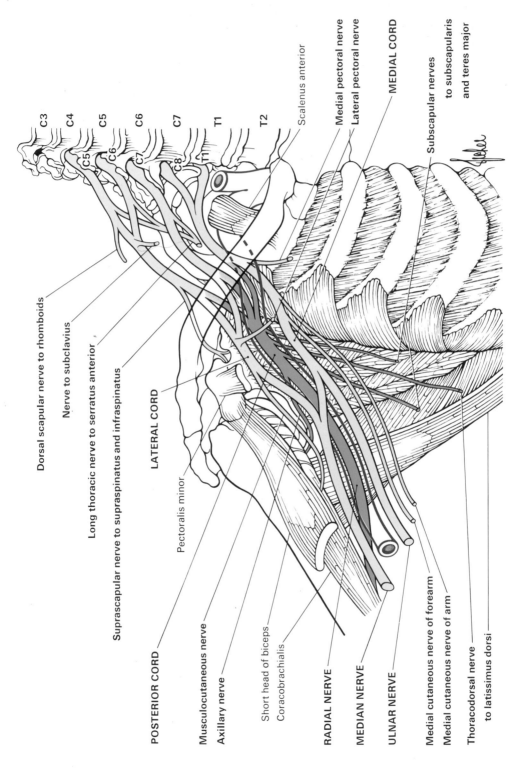

C3
C4
C5
C6
C7
T1
T2

C5
C6
C7
C8
T1

Scalenus anterior

Medial pectoral nerve
Lateral pectoral nerve

MEDIAL CORD

Subscapular nerves
to subscapularis
and teres major

Dorsal scapular nerve to rhomboids

Nerve to subclavius

Long thoracic nerve to serratus anterior

Suprascapular nerve to supraspinatus and infraspinatus

LATERAL CORD

Pectoralis minor

POSTERIOR CORD

Musculocutaneous nerve

Axillary nerve

Short head of biceps

Coracobrachialis

RADIAL NERVE

MEDIAN NERVE

ULNAR NERVE

Medial cutaneous nerve of forearm

Medial cutaneous nerve of arm

Thoracodorsal nerve
to latissimus dorsi

Fig. 3   Diagram of the brachial plexus, its branches and the muscles which they supply.

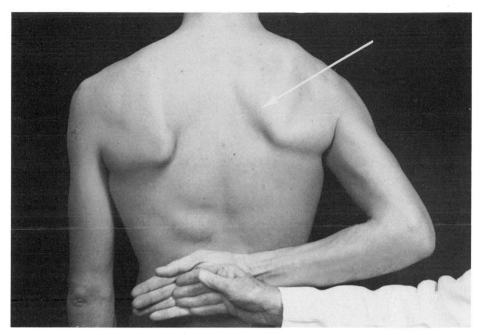

Fig. 4 Rhomboids (Dorsal scapular nerve; C4, C5)
The patient is pressing the palm of his hand backwards against the examiner's hand.
Arrow: the muscle bellies can be felt and sometimes seen.

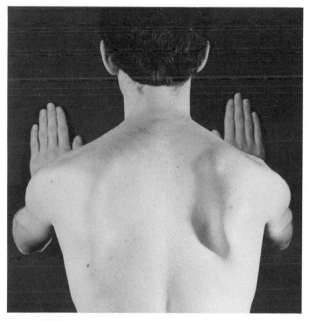

Fig. 5 Serratus anterior (Long thoracic nerve; C5, C6, C7)
The patient is pushing against a wall as in Fig. 2. The right serratus anterior is paralysed
and there is winging of the scapula.

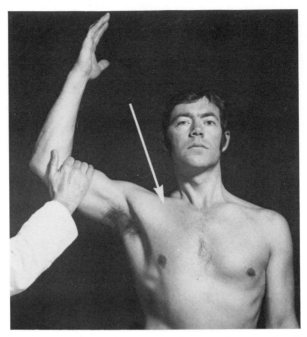

Fig. 6   Pectoralis Major: Clavicular Head (Lateral pectoral nerve; **C5,** C6)
The upper arm is above the horizontal and the patient is pushing forward against the examiner's hand. *Arrow:* the clavicular head of pectoralis major can be seen and felt.

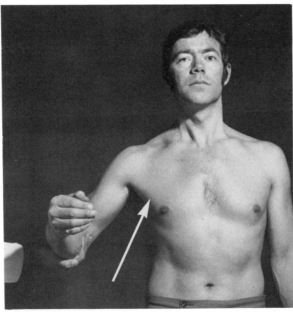

Fig. 7   Pectoralis Major: Sternocostal Head (Lateral and medial pectoral nerves; C6, **C7,** C8)
The patient is adducting the upper arm against resistance. *Arrow:* the sterno-costal head can be seen and felt.

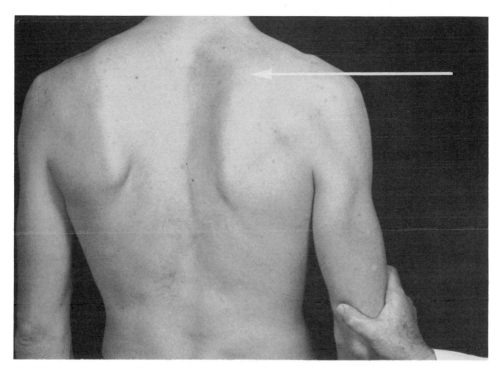

Fig. 8 Supraspinatus (Suprascapular nerve; **C5,** C6)
The patient is abducting the upper arm against resistance. *Arrow:* the muscle belly can be felt and sometimes seen.

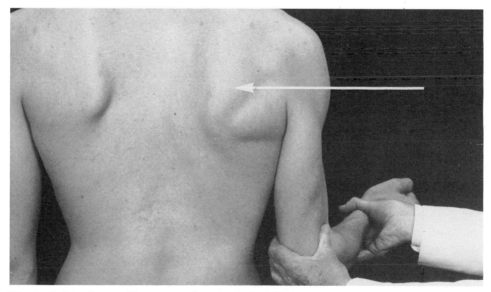

Fig. 9 Infraspinatus (Suprascapular nerve; **C5,** C6)
The patient is externally rotating the upper arm at the shoulder against resistance. The examiner's right hand is resisting the movement and supporting the forearm with the elbow at a right angle; his left hand is supporting the elbow and preventing abduction of the arm. *Arrow:* the muscle belly can be seen and felt.

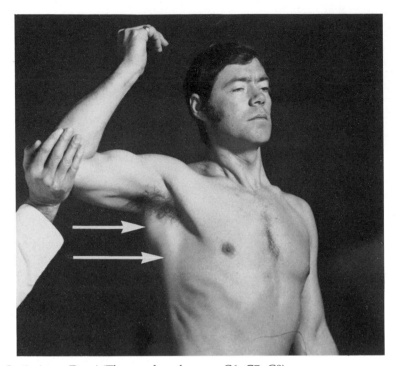

Fig. 10   Latissimus Dorsi (Thoracodorsal nerve; C6, **C7,** C8)
The upper arm is horizontal and the patient is adducting it against resistance.
Lower arrow: the muscle belly can be seen and felt. The upper arrow points to teres major.

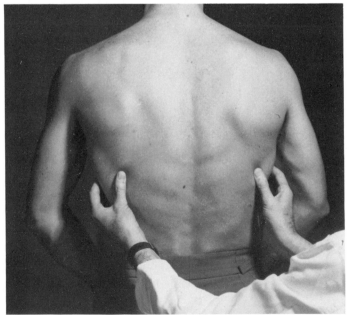

Fig. 11   Latissimus Dorsi (Thoracodorsal nerve; C6, **C7,** C8)
The muscle bellies can be felt to contract when the patient coughs.

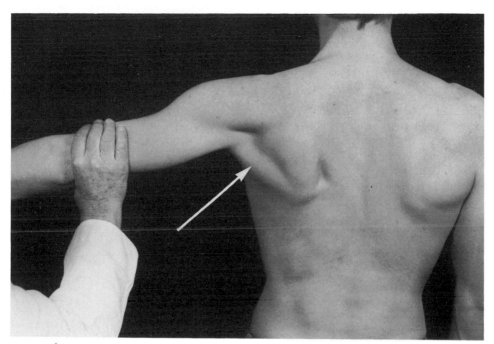

Fig. 12 Teres Major (Subscapular nerve; C5, C6, C7)
The patient is adducting the elevated upper arm against resistance. *Arrow:* the muscle belly can be seen and felt.

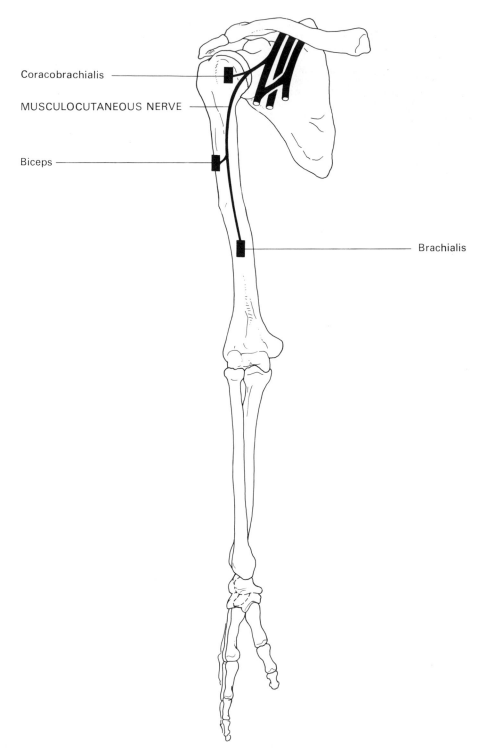

Coracobrachialis

MUSCULOCUTANEOUS NERVE

Biceps

Brachialis

Fig. 13   Diagram of the musculocutaneous nerve and the muscles which it supplies. (Modified from Pitres and Testut (1925) *Les Neufs en Schemas*, Doin, Paris.)

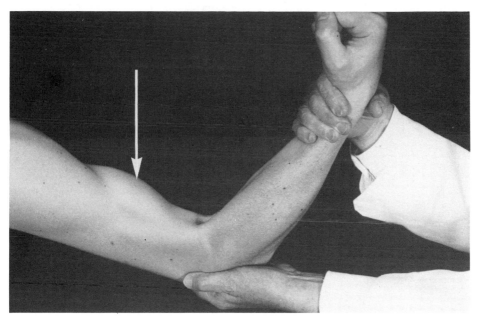

Fig. 14   Biceps (Musculocutaneous nerve; C5, C6)
The patient is flexing the supinated forearm against resistance. *Arrow:* the muscle belly can be seen and felt.

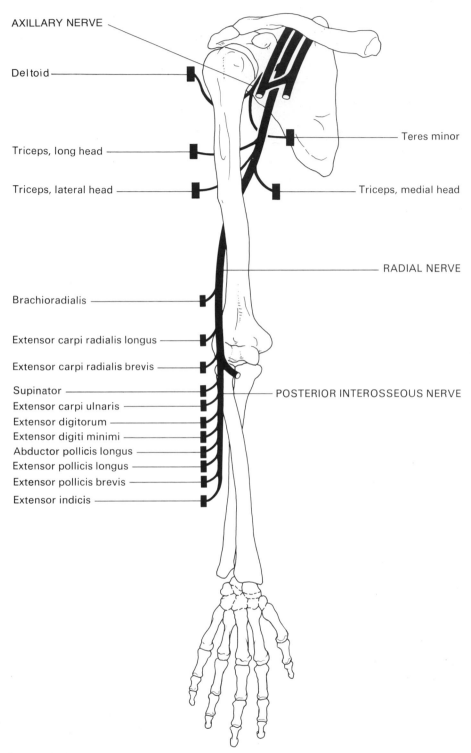

AXILLARY NERVE

Deltoid

Teres minor

Triceps, long head

Triceps, lateral head

Triceps, medial head

RADIAL NERVE

Brachioradialis

Extensor carpi radialis longus

Extensor carpi radialis brevis

Supinator

POSTERIOR INTEROSSEOUS NERVE

Extensor carpi ulnaris

Extensor digitorum

Extensor digiti minimi

Abductor pollicis longus

Extensor pollicis longus

Extensor pollicis brevis

Extensor indicis

Fig. 15   Diagram of the axillary and radial nerves and the muscles which they supply. (Modified from Pitres and Testut.)

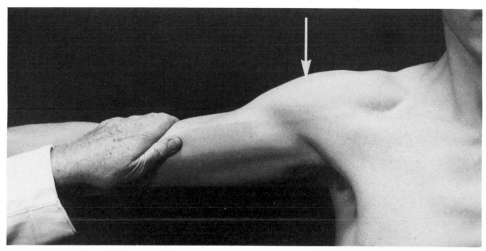

Fig. 16 Deltoid (Axillary nerve; **C5,** C6)
The patient is abducting the upper arm against resistance. *Arrow:* the anterior and middle fibres of the muscle can be seen and felt.

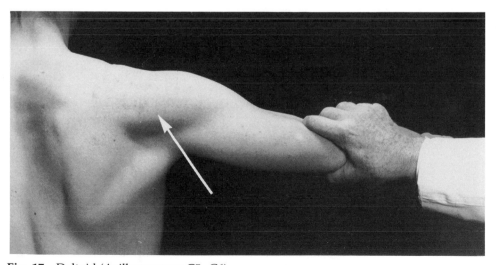

Fig. 17 Deltoid (Axillary nerve; **C5,** C6)
The patient is retracting the abducted upper arm against resistance. *Arrow:* the posterior fibres of deltoid can be seen and felt.

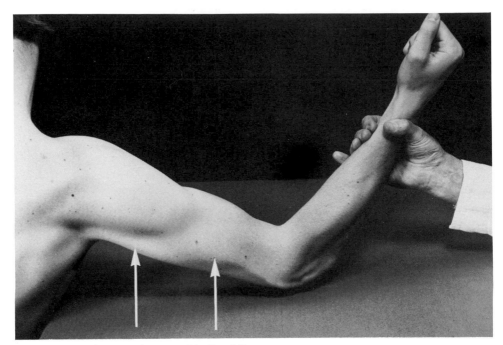

Fig. 18   Triceps (Radial nerve; C6, **C7,** C8)
The patient is extending the forearm at the elbow against resistance. The elbow is supported on a table. *Arrows:* the long and lateral heads of the muscle can be seen and felt.

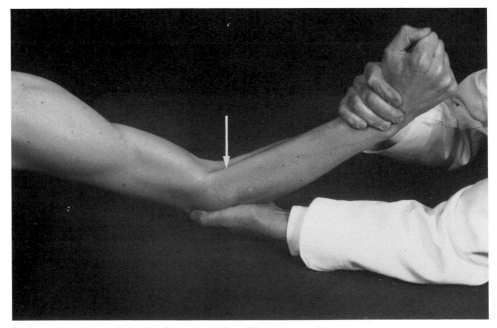

Fig. 19   Brachioradialis (Radial nerve; C5, **C6**)
The patient is flexing the forearm against resistance with the forearm midway between pronation and supination. *Arrow:* the muscle belly can be seen and felt.

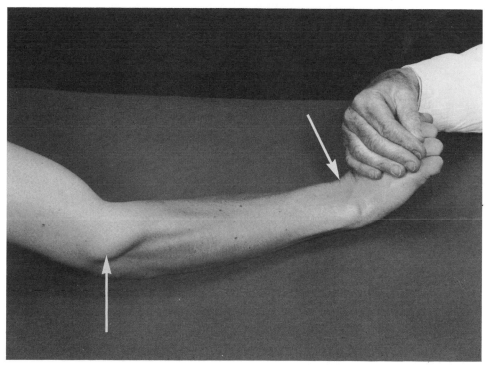

Fig. 20 Extensor Carpi Radialis Longus (Radial nerve; C5, **C6**)
The patient is extending and abducting the hand at the wrist against resistance.
Arrows: the muscle belly and tendon can be felt and usually seen.

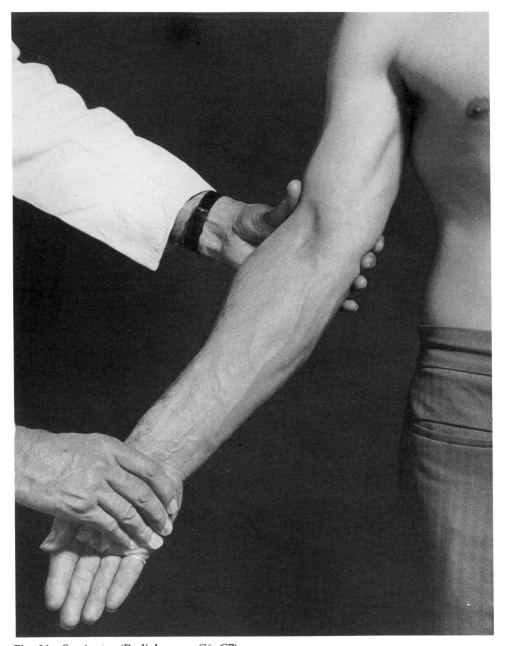

Fig. 21   Supinator (Radial nerve; C6, C7)
The patient is supinating the forearm against resistance with the forearm extended at the elbow.

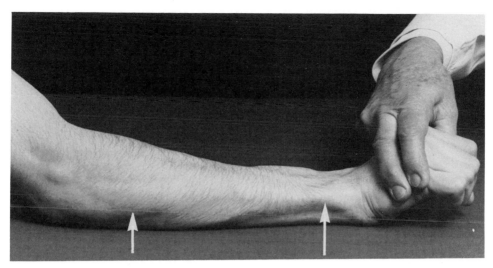

Fig. 22 Extensor Carpi Ulnaris (Posterior interosseous nerve; **C7, C8**)
The patient is extending and adducting the hand at the wrist against resistance.
Arrows: the muscle belly and the tendon can be seen and felt.

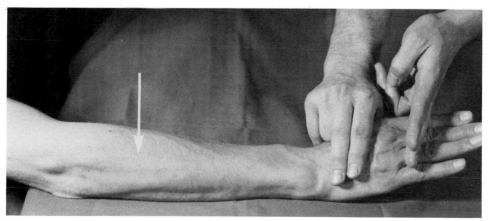

Fig. 23 Extensor Digitorum (Posterior interosseous nerve; **C7, C8**)
The patient's hand is firmly supported by the examiner's right hand. Extension at the
metacarpophalangeal joints is maintained against the resistance of the fingers of the
examiner's left hand. *Arrow:* the muscle belly can be seen and felt.

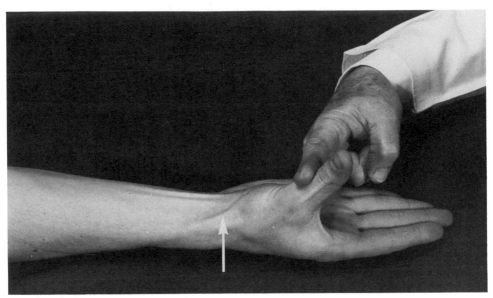

Fig. 24   Abductor Pollicis Longus (Posterior interosseous nerve; **C7**, C8)
The patient is abducting the thumb at the carpo-metacarpal joint in a plane at right angles to the palm. *Arrow:* the tendon can be seen and felt anterior and closely adjacent to the tendon of extensor pollicis brevis (**cf.** Fig. 26).

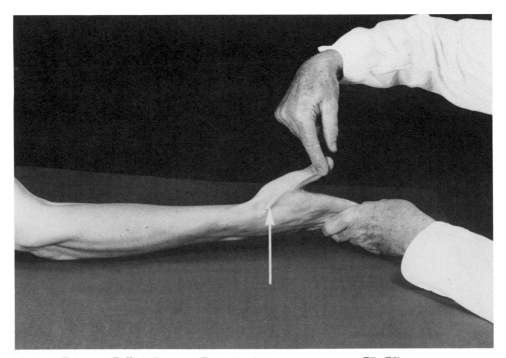

Fig. 25   Extensor Pollicis Longus (Posterior interosseous nerve; **C7**, C8)
The patient is extending the thumb at the interphalangeal joint against resistance.
Arrow: the tendon can be seen and felt.

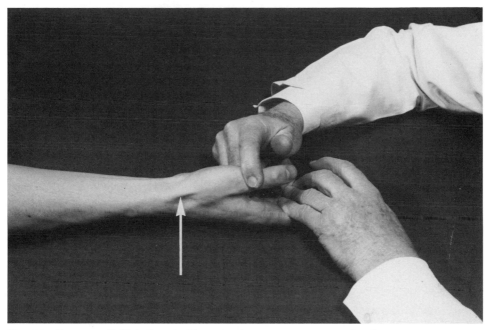

Fig. 26   Extensor Pollicis Brevis (Posterior interosseous nerve; **C7**, C8)
The patient is extending the thumb at the metacarpophalangeal joint against resistance.
Arrow: the tendon can be seen and felt (**cf.** Fig. 24).

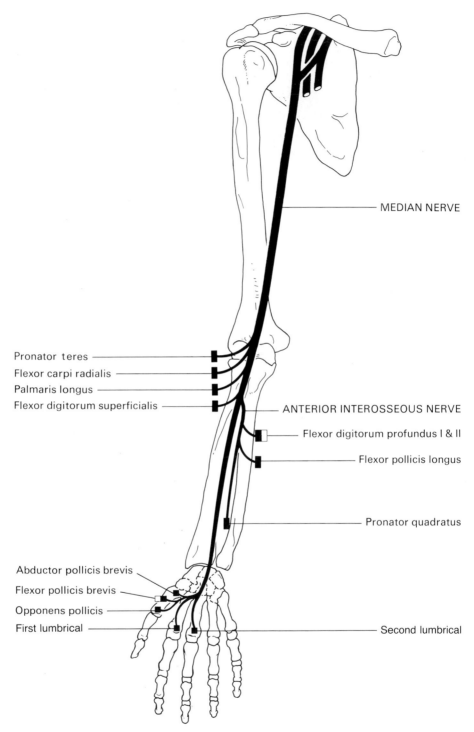

MEDIAN NERVE

Pronator teres

Flexor carpi radialis

Palmaris longus

Flexor digitorum superficialis

ANTERIOR INTEROSSEOUS NERVE

Flexor digitorum profundus I & II

Flexor pollicis longus

Pronator quadratus

Abductor pollicis brevis

Flexor pollicis brevis

Opponens pollicis

First lumbrical

Second lumbrical

Fig. 27 Diagram of the median nerve and the muscles which it supplies.
(Modified from Pitres and Testut.) Note: the white rectangle signifies that the muscle
indicated receives a part of its nerve supply from another peripheral nerve (**cf.** Figs. 36,
46 and 47).

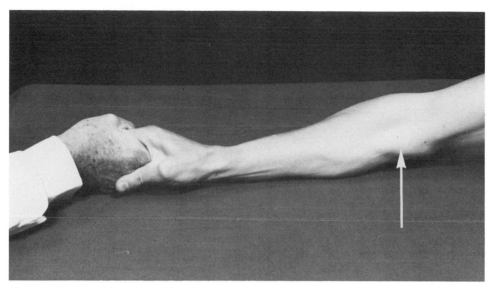

Fig. 28 Pronator Teres (Median nerve; C6, C7)
The patient is pronating the forearm against resistance. *Arrow:* the muscle belly can be felt and sometimes seen.

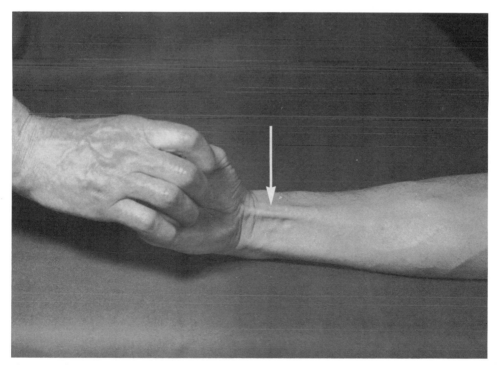

Fig. 29 Flexor Carpi Radialis (Median nerve; C6, C7)
The patient is flexing and abducting the hand at the wrist against resistance.
Arrow: the tendon can be seen and felt.

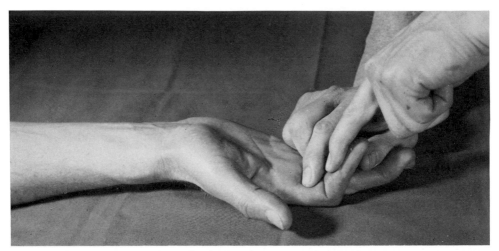

Fig. 30 Flexor Digitorum Superficialis (Median nerve; C7, **C8**, T1)
The patient is flexing the finger at the proximal interphalangeal joint against resistance with the proximal phalanx fixed. This test does not eliminate the possibility of flexion at the proximal interphalangeal joint being produced by flexor digitorum profundus.

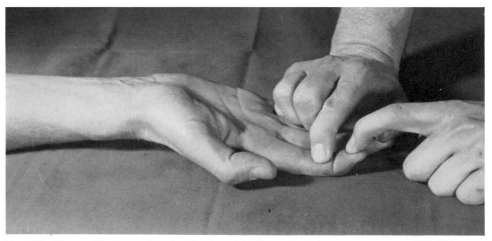

Fig. 31 Flexor Digitorum Profundus I and II (Anterior interosseous nerve; C7, **C8**)
The patient is flexing the distal phalanx of the index finger against resistance with the middle phalanx fixed.

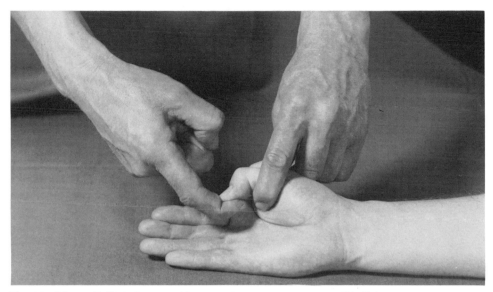

Fig. 32 Flexor Pollicis Longus (Anterior interosseous nerve; C7, **C8**)
The patient is flexing the distal phalanx of the thumb against resistance while the proximal phalanx is fixed.

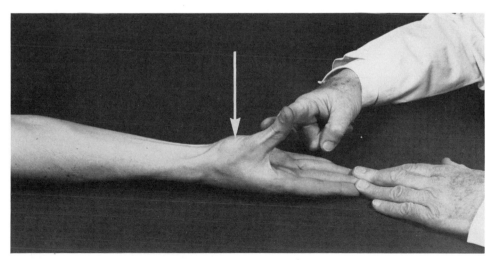

Fig. 33 Abductor Pollicis Brevis (Median nerve; C8, **T1**)
The patient is abducting the thumb at right angles to the palm against resistance.

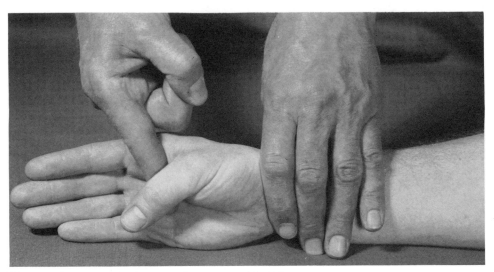

Fig. 34   Opponens Pollicis (Median nerve; C8, **T1**)
The patient is touching the base of the little finger with the thumb against resistance.

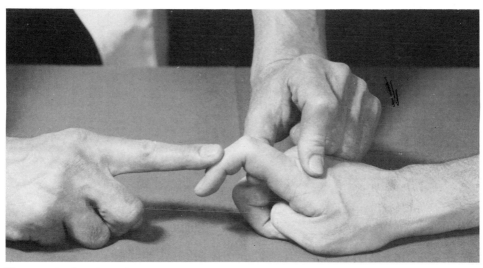

Fig. 35 1st Lumbrical-Interosseous Muscle (Median and ulnar nerves; C8, **T1**)
The patient is extending the finger at the proximal interphalangeal joint against resistance with the metacarpophalangeal joint hyperextended and fixed.

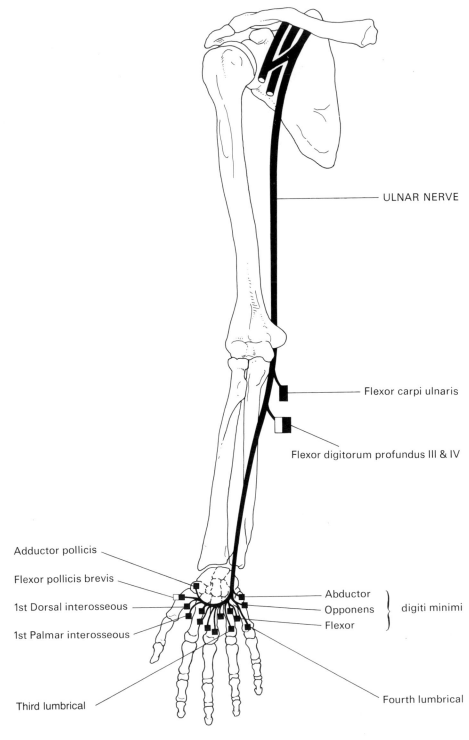

Fig. 36 Diagram of the ulnar nerve and the muscles which it supplies.
(Modified from Pitres and Testut.)

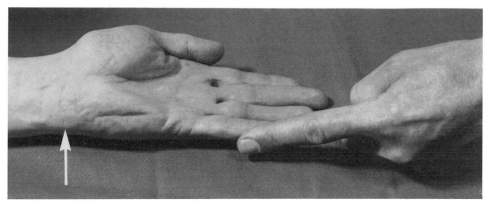

Fig. 37   Flexor Carpi Ulnaris (Ulnar nerve; C7, **C8,** T1)
The patient is abducting the little finger against resistance. The tendon of flexor carpi ulnaris can be seen and felt (arrow) as the muscle comes into action to fix the pisiform bone from which abductor digiti minimi arises. If flexor carpi ulnaris is intact, the tendon is seen even when abductor digiti minimi is paralysed (see also Fig. 38).

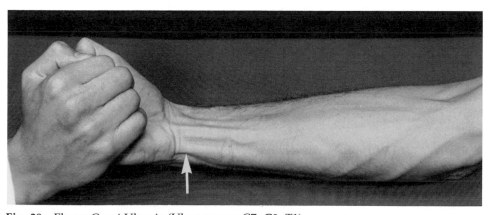

Fig. 38   Flexor Carpi Ulnaris (Ulnar nerve; C7, **C8,** T1)
The patient is flexing and adducting the hand at the wrist against resistance. *Arrow:* the tendon can be seen and felt.

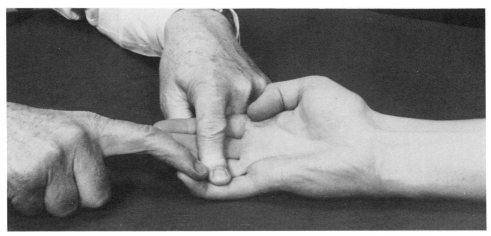

Fig. 39   Flexor Digitorum Profundus III and IV (Ulnar nerve; C7, **C8**)
The patient is flexing the distal interphalangeal joint against resistance while the middle phalanx is fixed.

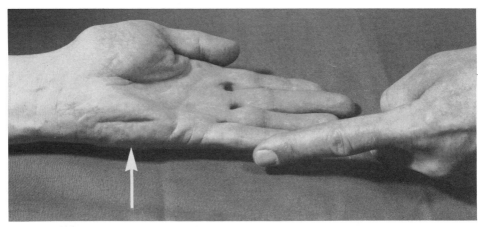

Fig. 40   Abductor Digiti Minimi (Ulnar nerve; **C8, T1**)
The back of the hand and fingers are flat upon the table. The patient is abducting the little finger against resistance. *Arrow:* the muscle belly can be felt and seen.

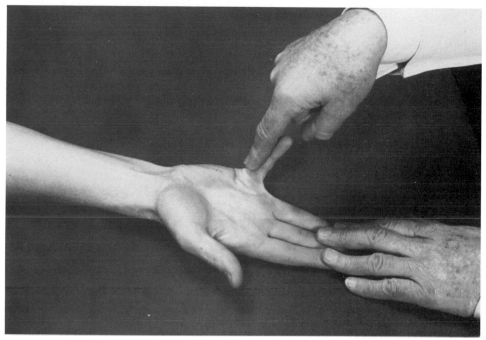

Fig. 41 Flexor Digiti Minimi (Ulnar nerve; C8, **T1**)
The patient is flexing the little finger at the metacarpophalangeal joint against resistance
with the interphalangeal joints held extended.

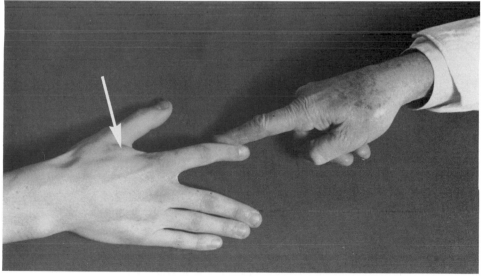

Fig. 42 First Dorsal Interosseous Muscle (Ulnar nerve; C8, **T1**)
The palm and fingers are flat upon a table. The patient is abducting the index finger
against resistance. *Arrow:* the muscle belly can be felt and usually seen.

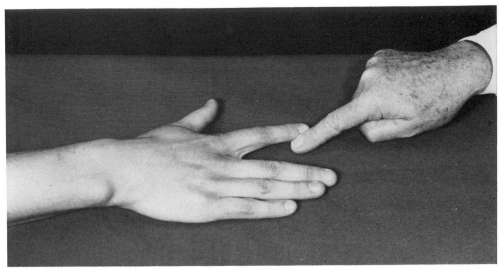

Fig. 43   Second Palmar Interosseous Muscle (Ulnar nerve; C8, **T1**)
The palm and fingers are flat upon a table. The patient is adducting the index finger against resistance.

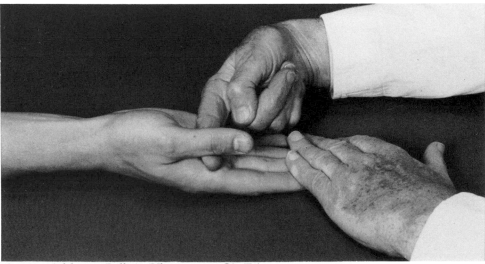

Fig. 44   Adductor Pollicis (Ulnar nerve; C8, **T1**)
The patient is adducting the thumb at right angles to the palm against the resistance of the examiner's finger.

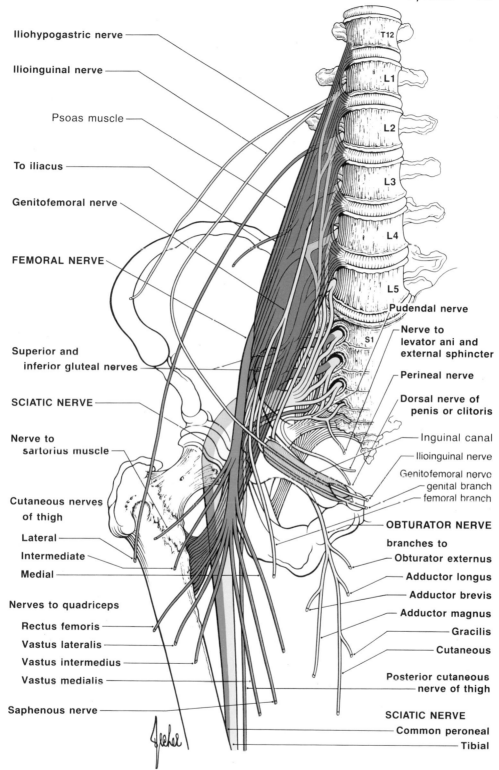

Fig. 45 Diagram of the lumbosacral plexus, its branches and the muscles which they supply.

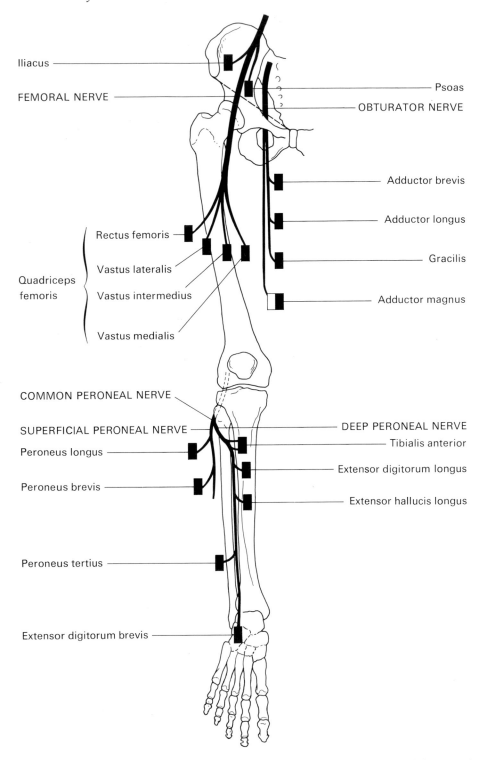

Iliacus

FEMORAL NERVE

Psoas

OBTURATOR NERVE

Adductor brevis

Adductor longus

Rectus femoris

Gracilis

Vastus lateralis

Quadriceps
femoris

Vastus intermedius

Adductor magnus

Vastus medialis

COMMON PERONEAL NERVE

SUPERFICIAL PERONEAL NERVE

DEEP PERONEAL NERVE

Tibialis anterior

Peroneus longus

Extensor digitorum longus

Peroneus brevis

Extensor hallucis longus

Peroneus tertius

Extensor digitorum brevis

Fig. 46   Diagram of the nerves on the anterior aspect of the lower limb, and the muscles which they supply. (Modified from Pitres and Testut.)

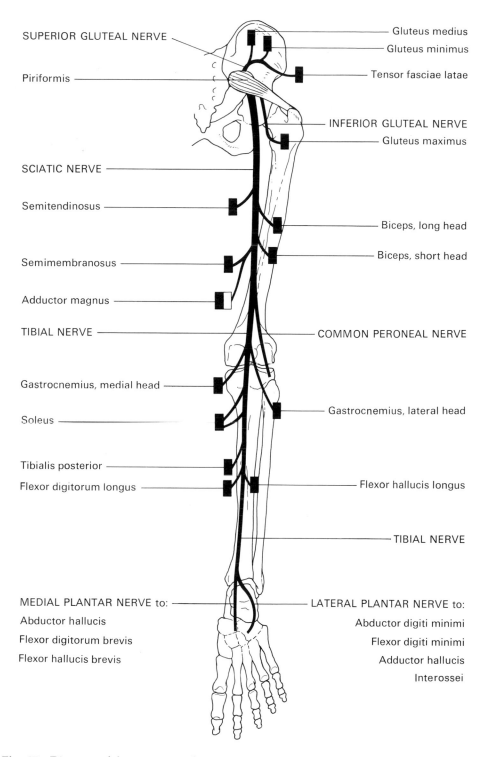

SUPERIOR GLUTEAL NERVE

Piriformis

SCIATIC NERVE

Semitendinosus

Semimembranosus

Adductor magnus

TIBIAL NERVE

Gastrocnemius, medial head

Soleus

Tibialis posterior

Flexor digitorum longus

MEDIAL PLANTAR NERVE to:
Abductor hallucis
Flexor digitorum brevis
Flexor hallucis brevis

Gluteus medius
Gluteus minimus

Tensor fasciae latae

INFERIOR GLUTEAL NERVE
Gluteus maximus

Biceps, long head

Biceps, short head

COMMON PERONEAL NERVE

Gastrocnemius, lateral head

Flexor hallucis longus

TIBIAL NERVE

LATERAL PLANTAR NERVE to:
Abductor digiti minimi
Flexor digiti minimi
Adductor hallucis
Interossei

Fig. 47 Diagram of the nerves on the posterior aspect of the lower limb, and the muscles which they supply. (Modified from Pitres and Testut.)

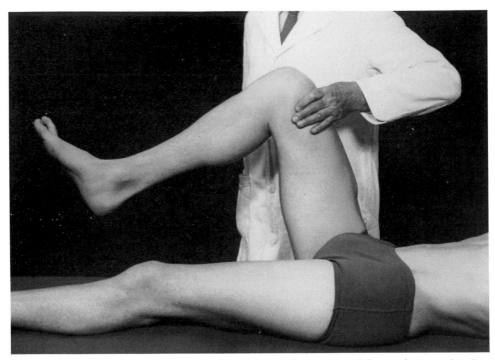

Fig. 48   Iliopsoas (Branches from L1, 2 and 3 spinal nerves and femoral nerve; **L1, L2,** L3)
The patient is flexing the thigh against resistance with the leg flexed at the knee and hip.

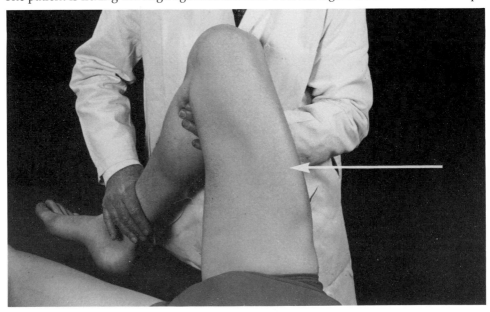

Fig. 49   Quadriceps Femoris (Femoral nerve; L2, **L3, L4**)
The patient is extending the leg against resistance with the limb flexed at the hip and knee. To detect slight weakness, the leg should be fully flexed at the knee. *Arrow:* the muscle belly of rectus femoris can be seen and felt.

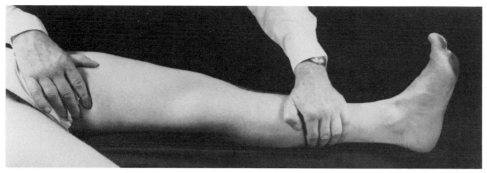

Fig. 50   Adductors (Obturator nerve; **L2, L3,** L4)
The patient lies on his back with the leg extended at the knee, and is adducting the limb against resistance. The muscle bellies can be felt.

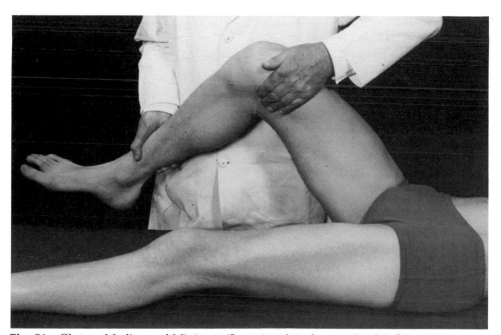

Fig. 51   Gluteus Medius and Minimus (Superior gluteal nerve; **L4, L5,** S1)
The patient lies on his back and is internally rotating the thigh against resistance with the limb flexed at the hip and knee.

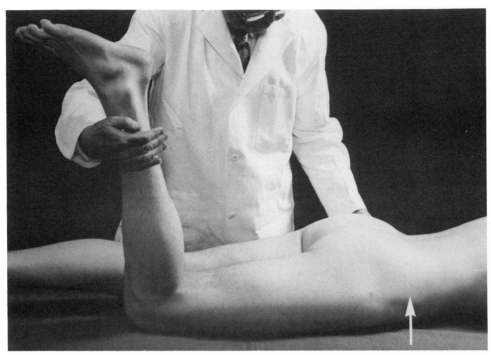

Fig. 52   Gluteus Medius and Minimus (Superior gluteal nerve; **L4, L5,** S1)
(An alternative method to that illustrated in Fig. 51.) The patient lies on his face with the leg flexed at the knee to a right angle and is internally rotating the limb against resistance. *Arrow:* the muscle bellies can be felt and sometimes seen.

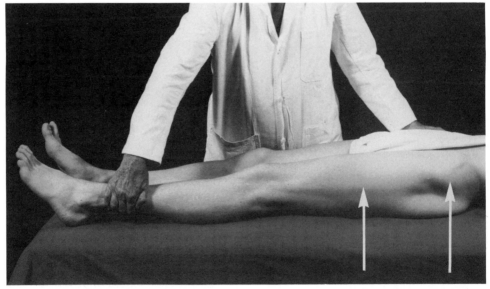

Fig. 53   Gluteus Medius and Minimus and Tensor Fasciae Latae (Superior gluteal nerve; **L4, L5,** S1)
The patient lies on his back with the leg extended and is abducting the limb against resistance. *Arrows:* the muscle bellies can be felt and sometimes seen.

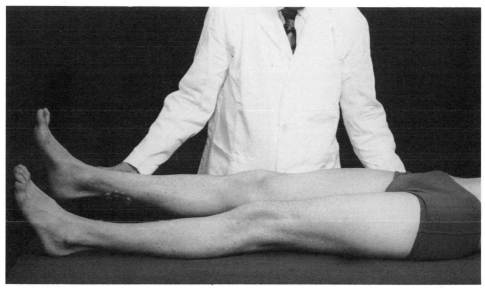

Fig. 54 Gluteus Maximus (Inferior gluteal nerve; **L5, S1,** S2)
The patient lies on his back with the leg extended at the knee and is extending the limb
at the hip against resistance. The examiner's left hand is feeling the muscle.

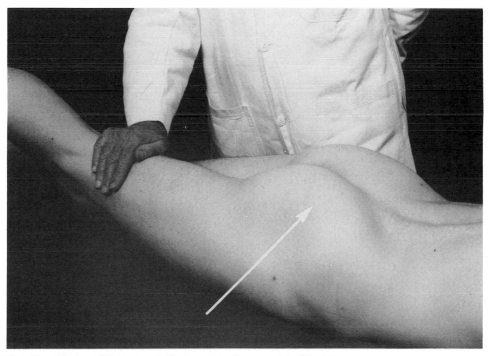

Fig. 55 Gluteus Maximus (Inferior gluteal nerve; **L5, S1,** S2)
The patient lies on his face and is elevating the leg against resistance. *Arrow:* the muscle
belly can be felt and often seen.

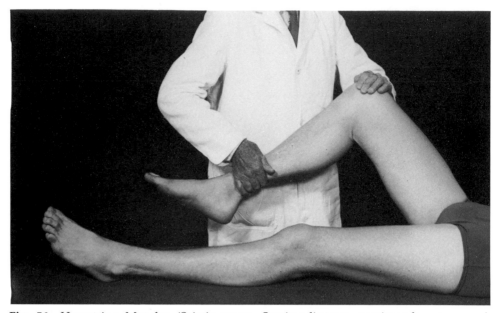

Fig. 56 Hamstring Muscles (Sciatic nerve. Semitendinosus, semimembranosus and biceps; L5, **S1,** S2)
The patient lies on his back with the limb flexed at the hip and knee and is flexing the leg at the knee against resistance.

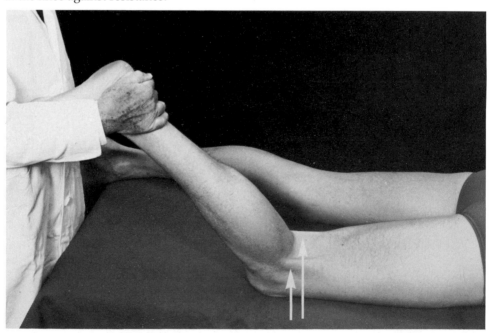

Fig. 57 Hamstring Muscles (Sciatic nerve. Semitendinosus, semimembranosus and biceps; L5, **S1,** S2)
The patient lies on his face and is flexing the leg at the knee against resistance. *Arrows:* the tendons of the biceps (laterally) and semitendinosus (medially) can be felt and usually seen.

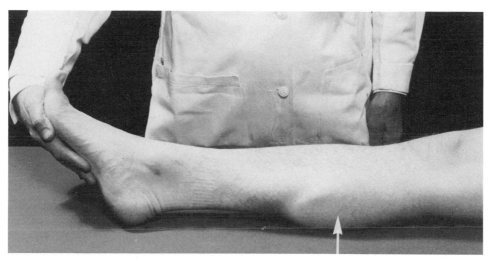

Fig. 58 Gastrocnemius (Tibial nerve; S1, S2)
The patient lies on his back with the leg extended and is plantar-flexing the foot against resistance. *Arrow:* the muscle bellies can be seen and felt. To detect slight weakness, the patient should be asked to stand on one foot, raise the heel from the ground and maintain this position.

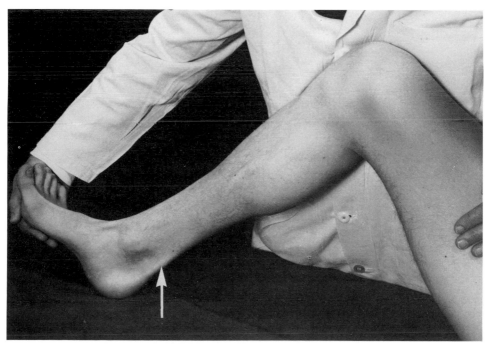

Fig. 59 Soleus (Tibial nerve; S1, S2)
The patient lies on his back with the limb flexed at the hip and knee and is plantar-flexing the foot against resistance. The muscle belly can be felt and sometimes seen. *Arrow:* the Achilles tendon.

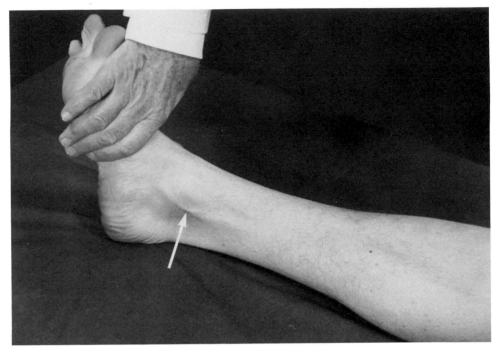

Fig. 60   Tibialis Posterior (Tibial nerve; L4, L5)
The patient is inverting the foot against resistance. *Arrow:* the tendon can be seen and felt.

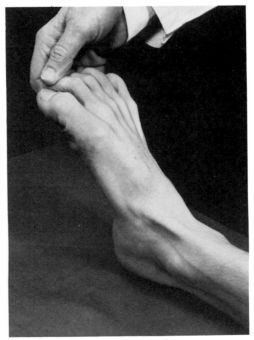

Fig. 61   Flexor Digitorum Longus, Flexor Hallucis Longus (Tibial nerve; L5, **S1, S2**)
The patient is flexing the toes against resistance.

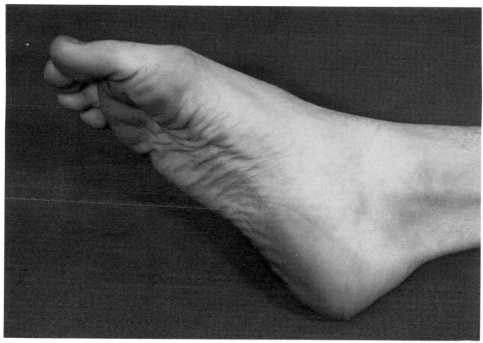

Fig. 62 Small muscles of the foot (medial and lateral plantar nerves; S1, S2)
The patient is cupping the sole of the foot; the small muscles can be felt and sometimes seen.

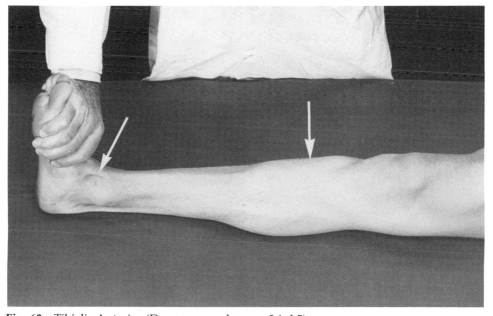

Fig. 63 Tibialis Anterior (Deep peroneal nerve; **L4,** L5)
The patient is dorsiflexing the foot against resistance. *Arrows:* the muscle belly and its tendon can be seen and felt.

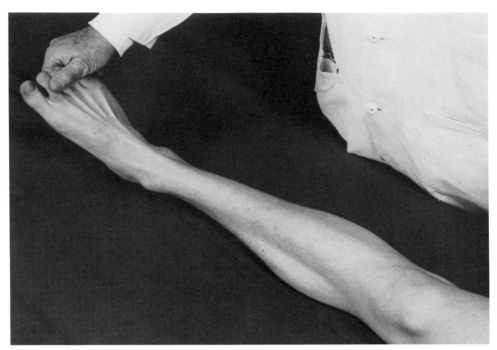

Fig. 64   Extensor Digitorum Longus (Deep peroneal nerve; **L5,** S1)
The patient is dorsiflexing the toes against resistance. The tendons passing to the lateral four toes can be seen and felt.

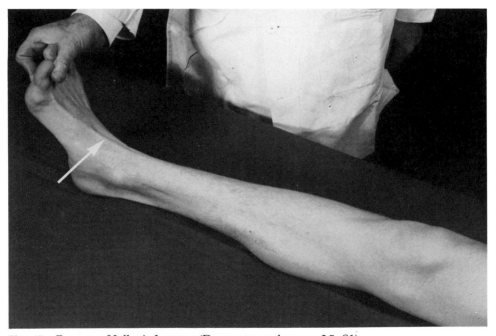

Fig. 65   Extensor Hallucis Longus (Deep peroneal nerve; **L5,** S1)
The patient is dorsiflexing the distal phalanx of the big toe against resistance. *Arrow:* the tendon can be seen and felt.

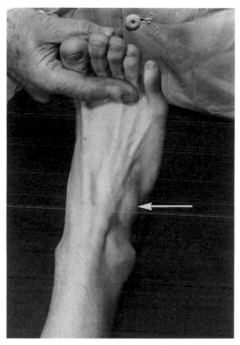

Fig. 66 Extensor Digitorum Brevis (Deep peroneal nerve; L5, S1)
The patient is dorsiflexing the proximal phalanges of the toes against resistance.
Arrow: the muscle belly can be felt and sometimes seen.

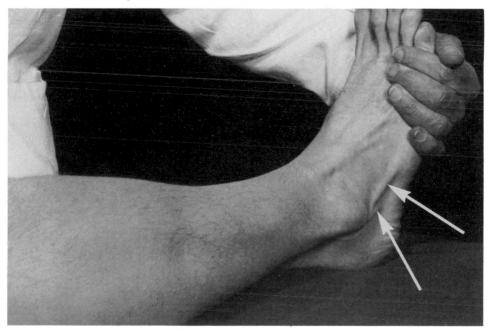

Fig. 67 Peroneus Longus and Brevis (Superficial peroneal nerve; L5, S1)
The patient is everting the foot against resistance. *Upper arrow:* the tendon of peroneus
brevis. *Lower arrow:* the tendon of peroneus longus.

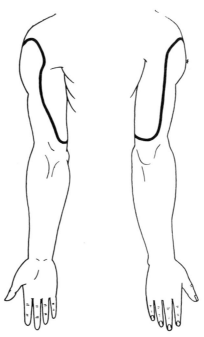

Fig. 68 The approximate area within which sensory changes may be found in complete lesions of the brachial plexus (C5, C6, C7, C8, T1).

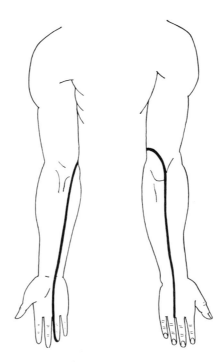

Fig. 69 The approximate area within which sensory changes may be found in lesions of the lower roots (C8, T1) of the brachial plexus.

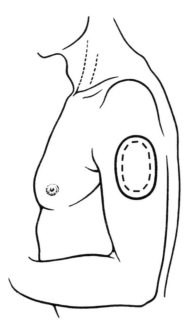

Fig. 70   The approximate area within which sensory changes may be found in lesions of the axillary nerve. Light touch, continuous line; pin-prick, dotted line.

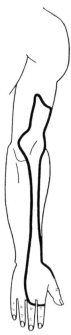

Fig. 71   The approximate area within which sensory changes may be found in high lesions of the radial nerve (above the origin of the posterior cutaneous nerves of the arm and forearm). The average area is usually considerably smaller, and absence of sensory changes has been recorded.

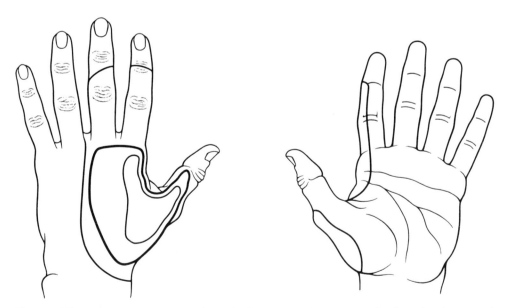

Fig. 72   The approximate area within which sensory changes may be found in lesions of the radial nerve above the elbow joint and below the origin of the posterior cutaneous nerve of the forearm. (The distribution of the superficial terminal branch of the radial nerve.) Heavy line, average area; light lines, small and large areas.

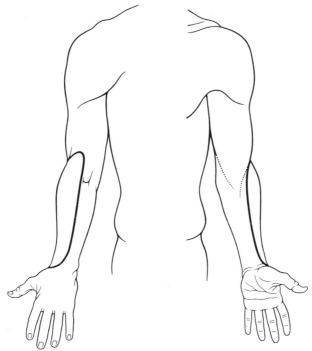

Fig. 73 The approximate area within which sensory changes may be found in lesions of the musculocutaneous nerve. (The distribution of the lateral cutaneous nerve of the forearm.)

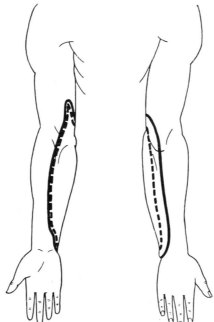

Fig. 74 The approximate area within which sensory changes may be found in lesions of the medial cutaneous nerve of the forearm. Light touch, continuous line; pin-prick, dotted line.

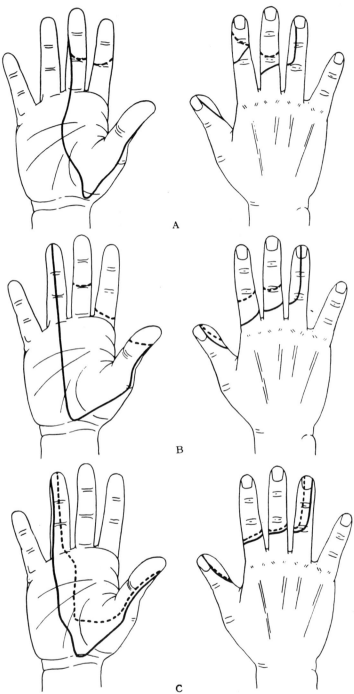

Fig. 75 The approximate areas within which sensory changes may be found in lesions of the median nerve. A = small area, B = average area, and C = large area. Light touch, continuous line; pin-prick, dotted line. Immediately after complete division of the median nerve, the insensitive area on the palm of the hand may be somewhat larger than is shown. (Modified from Head and Sherren (1905) *Brain,* **28,** 116.)

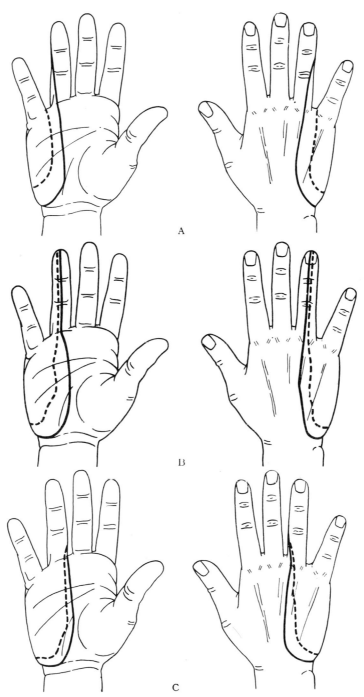

Fig. 76 The approximate areas within which sensory changes may be found in lesions of the ulnar nerve. A = small area, B = average area, and C = large area. Light touch, continuous line; pin-prick, dotted line. Immediately after complete division of the ulnar nerve, the insensitive area on the palm of the hand may be somewhat larger than is shown. (Modified from Head and Sherren.)

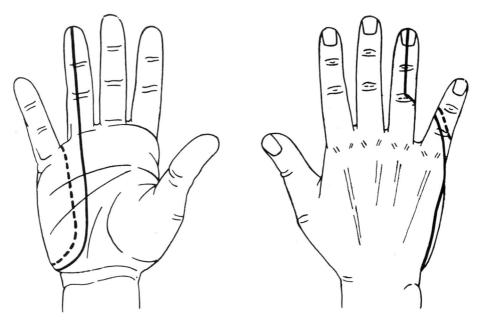

Fig. 77   The approximate area within which sensory changes may be found in lesions of the ulnar nerve below the origin of its dorsal branch. Light touch, continuous line; pinprick, dotted line. (Modified from Head and Sherren.)

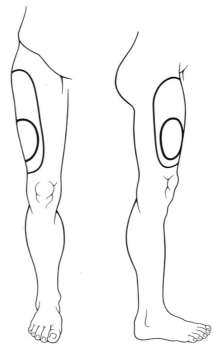

Fig. 78   The approximate area within which sensory changes may be found in lesions of the lateral cutaneous nerve of the thigh. Average area, heavy line; large area, light line.

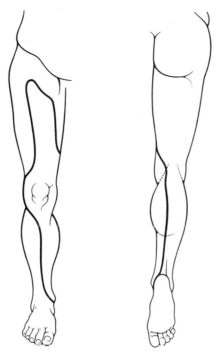

Fig. 79   The approximate area within which sensory changes may be found in lesions of the femoral nerve. (The distribution of the intermediate and medial cutaneous nerve of the thigh and the saphenous nerve.)

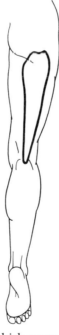

Fig. 80   The approximate area within which sensory changes may be found in lesions of the posterior cutaneous nerve of the thigh.

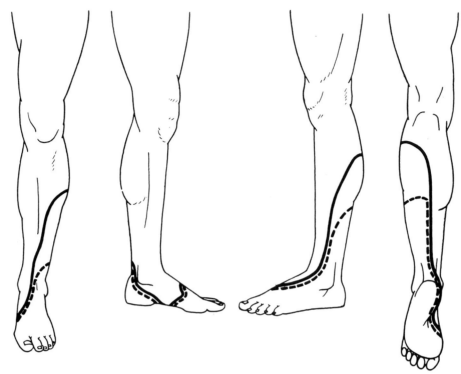

Fig. 81   The approximate area within which sensory changes may be found in lesions of the trunk of the sciatic nerve. Light touch, continuous line; pin-prick, dotted line. (Modified from M.R.C. Special Report No. 54, 1920.)

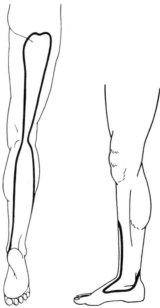

Fig. 82   The approximate area within which sensory changes may be found in lesions of both the sciatic and the posterior cutaneous nerve of the thigh.

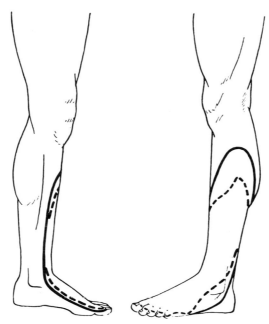

Fig. 83   The approximate area within which sensory changes may be found in lesions of the common peroneal nerve above the origin of the superficial peroneal nerve. Light touch, continuous line; pin-prick, dotted line. (Modified from M.R.C. Special Report No. 54, 1920.)

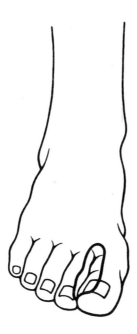

Fig. 84   The approximate area within which sensory changes may be found in lesions of the deep peroneal nerve.

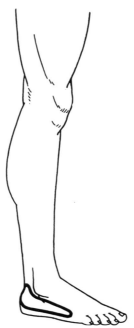

Fig. 85   The approximate area within which sensory changes may be found in lesions of the sural nerve.

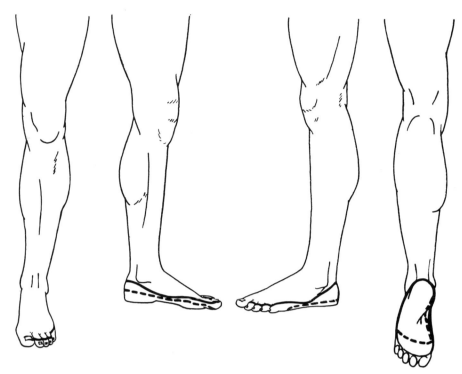

Fig. 86   The approximate area within which sensory changes may be found in lesions of the tibial nerve. Light touch, continuous line; pin-prick, dotted line. (Modified from M.R.C. Special Report No. 54, 1920.)

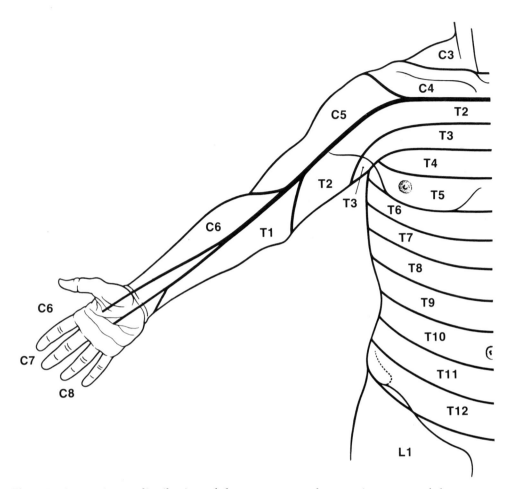

Fig. 87 Approximate distribution of dermatomes on the anterior aspect of the upper limb.

Fig. 87–90 show the approximate cutaneous areas supplied by each spinal root. There is considerable variation and overlap between dermatomes so that an isolated root lesion results in a much smaller area of sensory impairment than is indicated in these diagrams.

This variation also applies to the innervation of the fingers, but the thumb is usually supplied by C6 and the little finger usually by C8 (see Inouye and Buchthal (1977) *Brain* **100:** 731–748).

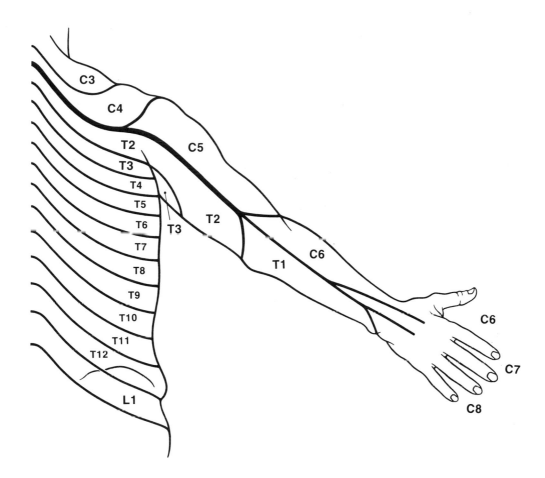

Fig. 88 Approximate distribution of dermatomes on the posterior aspect of the upper limb.

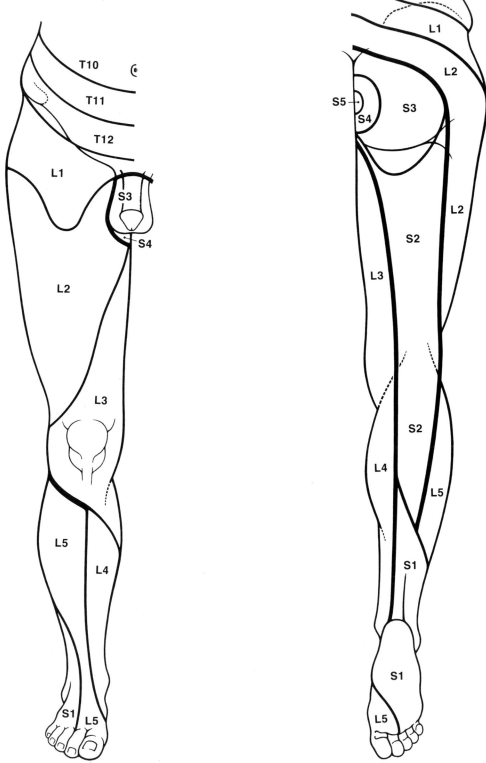

Fig. 89   Approximate distribution of dermatomes on the lower limb.

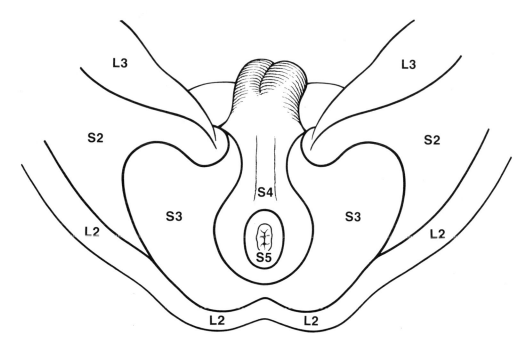

Fig. 90 Approximate distribution of dermatomes on the perineum.

Nerve and main root supply of muscles
(The list given below does not include all the muscles innervated by these nerves, but only those more commonly tested, either clinically or electrically, and shows the order of innervation.)

Upper Limb	Spinal Roots
Spinal Accessory Nerve	
Trapezius	C3, C4
Brachial Plexus	
Rhomboids	C4, C5
Serratus anterior	C5, C6, C7
Pectoralis major	
Clavicular	**C5**, C6
Sternal	C6, **C7**, C8
Supraspinatus	**C5**, C6
Infraspinatus	**C5**, C6
Latissimus dorsi	C6, **C7**, C8
Teres major	C5, C6, C7
Axillary Nerve	
Deltoid	**C5**, C6
Musculocutaneous Nerve	
Biceps	C5, C6
Brachialis	C5, C6
Radial Nerve	
Triceps { Long head / Lateral head / Medial head }	C6, **C7**, C8
Brachioradialis	C5, **C6**
Extensor carpi radialis longus	C5, **C6**
Posterior Interosseous Nerve	
Supinator	C6, C7
Extensor carpi ulnaris	**C7**, C8
Extensor digitorum	**C7**, C8
Abductor pollicis longus	**C7**, C8
Extensor pollicis longus	**C7**, C8
Extensor pollicis brevis	**C7**, C8
Extensor indicis	**C7**, C8
Median Nerve	
Pronator teres	C6, C7
Flexor carpi radialis	C6, C7
Flexor digitorum superficialis	C7, **C8**, T1
Abductor pollicis brevis	C8, **T1**
Flexor pollicis brevis*	C8, **T1**
Opponens pollicis	C8, **T1**
Lumbricals I & II	C8, **T1**

Anterior Interosseous Nerve
Pronator quadratus   C7, **C8**
Flexor digitorum profundus I & II   C7, **C8**
Flexor pollicis longus   C7, **C8**

Ulnar Nerve
Flexor carpi ulnaris   C7, **C8**, T1
Flexor digitorum profundus III & IV   C7, **C8**
Hypothenar muscles   C8, **T1**
Adductor pollicis   C8, **T1**
Flexor pollicis brevis   C8, **T1**
Palmar interossei   C8, **T1**
Dorsal interossei   C8, **T1**
Lumbricals III & IV   C8, **T1**

Lower Limb	Spinal Roots

Femoral Nerve
Iliopsoas   **L1, L2**, L3
Rectus femoris ⎫
Vastus lateralis ⎪ Quadriceps
Vastus intermedius ⎬ femoris   L2, **L3, L4**
Vastus medialis ⎭

Obturator Nerve
Adductor longus ⎫
Adductor magnus ⎭   **L2, L3**, L4

Superior Gluteal Nerve
Gluteus medius and minimus ⎫
Tensor fasciae latae ⎭   **L4, L5**, S1

Inferior Gluteal Nerve
Gluteus maximus   **L5, S1**, S2

Sciatic and Tibial Nerves
Semitendinosus   L5, **S1**, S2
Biceps   L5, **S1**, S2
Semimembranosus   L5, **S1**, S2
Gastrocnemius and soleus   S1, S2
Tibialis posterior   L4, L5
Flexor digitorum longus   L5, **S1, S2**
Abductor hallucis ⎫
Abductor digiti minimi ⎬ Small muscles   S1, S2
Interossei ⎭ of foot

Sciatic and Common Peroneal Nerves
Tibialis anterior   **L4**, L5
Extensor digitorum longus   **L5**, S1
Extensor hallucis longus   **L5**, S1
Extensor digitorum brevis   L5, S1
Peroneus longus   L5, S1
Peroneus brevis   L5, S1

*Flexor pollicis brevis is often supplied wholly or partially by the ulnar nerve.